Alzheimer's, healthy lifestyles and Mediterranean diet

Alzheimer's, Healthy Lifestyles And Mediterranean Diet

Gianni Perilli

GP Dementia Services New York, Inc.
Caregivercare

This book does not replace the advice of trained health professional. If you know or suspect that you have health problem, you should consult a health professional. The author and the publisher specifically disclaim any liability, loss or risk, personal or otherwise, that is incurred as a consequence, directly or indirectly, of the use and application of any the contents of this book.

ISBN-13: 978-0-692-13526-6

Published by:
GP Dementia Services New York, Inc.
170 East 88th Street, #2c
New York, New York 10128

To order: info@caregivercare.org

www.caregivercare.org

To those willing to preserve their mind

Table of Contents

Acknowledgments

I thank Mr. Michael Fisch. His generosity allowed the printing of this book.

I thank Dina Julsen, supportive friend. She always believed in the goodness of this initiative.

I thank Mr. Stefano M., a real expert about healthy foods.

I thank Lisa Zaccaria for her time and understanding.

From the bottom of my heart, I thank Pamela Downing for finicky proofreading and patient help in revising the draft.

I would like to thank Father Madigan, Mrs. Margaret Peet, all volunteers and good people I met at Saint Thomas More Church. They heartily collaborated to provide programs for our lovely seniors.

I thank God for putting in me the passion to study and to experience many things needed to try to help those who really want to preserve their mind, regardless of their age or their mental condition.

Foreword

Having served as a priest in the Archdiocese of New York for almost fifty years, I have had the opportunity on any number of occasions to engage families when one of their loved ones becomes beset by the symptoms of dementia with the onset of Alzheimer's disease. As people are able to live longer and longer, the downside of this blessing of living to a ripe old age is that that more and more people are becoming susceptible to the diminishment or loss of their cognitive abilities. This is, of course, a tragedy for the person afflicted with the disease. It is also a tragedy for the whole family, as they see someone who previously had appeared so vital, so energetic and so competent in all aspects of life slowly disappear into another world. Physically present, but mentally miles away, families struggle—some success-fully, other not—in meeting the challenges of the moment, in trying to provide a context of safety, of reassurance, of support for their afflicted family member.

It has been said (Hannah Arendt) that a society is only as strong as its members who can be trusted to remain faithful to the promises they have made. In that light, spouses come to learn the profound significance of the marriage vows that they uttered decades earlier when they promised to support their new wife or husband "in good times or in bad, in sickness and in health". Sons and daughters are given the opportunity to return to a helpless parent the care that they themselves received when they were helpless infants. Friends must decide whether they will continue to maintain the bonds of affection and conviviality that were forged in happier times. It is a time of decision—a time for those who profess themselves to be disciples of Jesus Christ to enter more deeply into the mystery of His death and resurrection, to carry the cross (For what is the cross but that which life throws at us, without our asking for it?), coming to know the joy and satisfaction of what it is to serve one who is so vulnerable.

Medical science is still trying to discover the causes and remedies for Alzheimer's disease. In the meanwhile, those of us who are not medical professionals often experience a sense of powerless and/or fatigue. Still we should not feel we are helpless, that there is nothing we can do. That is why I was delighted when Dr. Gianni Perilli established a program in the parish of which I am currently pastor, the Church of Our Lady of Good Counsel-St. Thomas More, in the Upper East Side of New York City, to support the caregivers of those suffering the symptoms of dementia, and to enable seniors in a variety of activities in maintaining their cognitive abilities. I have personally witnessed the delight with which they speak about the new worlds that have been opened to them, whether it be in learning a new language, in discovering how to communicate with faraway family members through the internet, in practicing new physical exercises, and in finding healthier ways to improve their diet. My hope is that what Dr. Perilli has developed in this setting might be a model for many others.

New York, May 30th 2018

Rev. Kevin V. Madigan, Pastor

xii

I

ALZHEIMER'S

Alzheimer's and dementia

What is the difference between Alzheimer's and dementia?

Alzheimer's is a disease; dementia is a list of symptoms. The two main types of symptoms in dementia are cognitive and behavioral.

Cognitive symptoms, in the first stage, would include such things as the inability to perform mathematical calculations correctly, or to remember events that have occurred, or to re-call the name of a person the Alzheimer's sufferer meets. First stage behavioral symptoms could include a strong sense of restlessness, giving up hobbies that the patient always had, or the first episodes of a personality change.

Alzheimer's causes dementia. The cause-effect relation exist-ing between Alzheimer's and dementia symptoms is like pneumonia and a cough: Alzheimer's and pneumonia are causes, dementia and a cough are effects.

Alzheimer's is only one of many possible diseases causing dementia. Not less than 50 types of diseases cause dementia, but the most common of these diseases are Alzheimer's, vascular dementia, Lewy body dementia, front temporal dementia, progressive supranuclear paralysis, Huntington's chorea and Parkinson's. Only one patient in three with Parkinson's shows dementia symptoms. Two out of three patients with dementia have Alzheimer's disease or Vascular dementia, these being the two most frequent diseases causing dementia.

Scientific literature studies utilize many different scales, sequencing the stages of symptoms in many different ways. Many scales start with Mild Cognitive Impairment (MCI) and end with final stage. "*MCI is an intermediate stage between the expected cognitive decline of normal aging and the more serious decline of dementia. It can involve problems with memory, language, thinking and judgment that are greater than normal age-related changes*".[1] A person affected by MCI is not yet considered a person suffering from dementia. Around 20% of people with MCI can reverse the symptoms.

Here follows a possible way to classify different clinical characteristics in dementia, from the beginning to the final stage. A person with one of these symptoms may not be diagnosed with Alzheimer's. And a person with one of these symptoms will not necessarily have all these symptoms.

---

[1] Mayo Clinic Staff. (1998-2018). Mild Cognitive impairment (MCI). Retrieved from https://www.mayoclinic.org/diseases-conditions/mild-cognitive-impairment/symptoms-causes/syc-20354578

2

Clinical characteristics[2]

As the disease advances, a person with Alzheimer's will move through a deepening succession of symptoms: The person may

1. several times, not be able to find the correct word for objects, or theoretical concepts in the company of friends and family.
2. lose and/or misplace objects many times and may blame others for taking them.
3. often have poor interactions when meeting with people in public settings and start to have some early problems with a lack of concentration.
4. have mild and moderate attacks of anxiety.
5. have a decreased knowledge about recent and current events.
6. have a decreased ability to remember events from his personal history.
7. have difficulty doing simple mathematical problems.
8. always deny that anything is wrong, in the absence of a diagnosis.
9. avoid challenging situations by gradually withdrawing.
10. have symptoms of depression.
11. have problems driving and traveling.
12. have difficulty handling financial issues and doing related calculations.
13. have a decreased ability to carry out more complex tasks.
14. have problems eating or drinking.

---

[2] Perilli, G. (2008). *Dementia Diary*. Washington, DC, USA. Copyright Library of Congress

15. deny problems that are evident, even after diagnosis.
16. be unable to remember the main aspects of daily life, recent events or recent experiences.
17. be confused about place.
18. be confused about time.
19. have difficulty choosing what clothes to wear.
20. have problems with bathroom activities.
21. have episodes of seizures.
22. have problems walking and standing up.
23. have difficulties speaking and communicating.
24. have a very superficial knowledge of his/her past life.
25. have some incidents of incontinence.
26. Have problems with insomnia and/or his/her sleep/wake cycle.
27. exhibit changes in feelings and emotions.
28. show a change in personality.
29. no longer be able to differentiate strangers from his/her relatives.
30. have hallucinations, deliriums, and delusions.
31. have excessive attachments.
32. have severe attacks of anxiety and often be agitated.
33. have violent and disproportionate behaviors that he/she never had in the past.
34. have lost the ability to communicate verbally.
35. now be incontinent.
36. be incapable of self feeding.
37. be unable to carry out bathroom activities without assistance.
38. have lost his/her psychomotor skills.
39. have decubitus ulcers (bedsores) and/or involuntary muscular contractions.

What happens in the brain when you have Alzheimer's?

In the brain of person with Alzheimer's disease who shows dementia symptoms three things can happen:

1) An abnormal accumulation of a protein, called beta-amyloid, makes plaques, which accrue in the synapses between brain cells. The neurons cannot communicate each other anymore.

2) An abnormal accumulation of another protein, called Tau, makes tangles, within nerve cells and choke the cell's nutrient transport, thus killing the cell.

3) An inflammation of neurons.

Fascinating studies report that some people, aged 80 to 100, whose autopsies revealed Alzheimer's levels of abundant tangles and plaque, never showed dementia symptoms. In these persons' brains, the immune systems had not reacted with the inflammatory response.

The brain starts not working properly anymore. Alzheimer's disease starts to defraud a person of his/her identity, robbing who he/she is, and over the years relatives see changes in the person they love. Whoever takes care of a loved one with the disease, knows very well that there is nothing more devastating than this.

Is Alzheimer's, or dementia, preventable?

Brain imaging studies reveal that the abnormal accumulation of the proteins tau and beta-amyloid starts from ten to twenty years before individuals show early symptoms. This seems similar to the relationship between cholesterol and heart attack: cholesterol starts to deposit in arteries years before the heart attack happens. The analogy, though, is limited. Cardiologists can use a pharmacological intervention to prevent heart attacks, like statins. After a heart attack, they also have effective medical treatments. Unfortunately, today doctors have no pharmacological interventions either to prevent dementia or to cure it.

However neuroscientists say that some non-pharmacological interventions can prevent and slow down the abnormal accumulation of these proteins. This means if people who are turning 45 start right now to follow these non-pharmacological interventions, they will benefit from them later on.

Is Alzheimer's disease curable?

Unfortunately, although Alzheimer's is treatable, it is not curable: The Food and Drug Administration (FDA) has approved five different drugs. These drugs treat only symptoms (symptomatic drugs). They do not cure the disease because they are not able to remove the cause. Persons diagnosed with cancer are treated and often cured; a person suffering from Alzheimer's can barely be treated and never cured.

The scientific community made huge breakthroughs in the treatment of cancer, HIV, heart attack and stroke in the last century. But if we look at scientific research on Alzheimer's, it is different. In 1901, a German woman had delusions and she could not remember even the most important and recent events of her life. Her doctor's name was Alzheimer and this woman was the first person in medical history diagnosed with the disease later called Alzheimer's disease. If this woman were alive today she could no more have pharmacological treatment for that disease than she had 117 years ago.

Underline At what age do Alzheimer's symptoms first appear?

Around 90%-95% of patients with Alzheimer's disease or other dementia are over 65 years old. Early signs of Alzheimer's disease start very slowly and gradually, almost imperceptibly at the beginning.

Roughly 10% of the population over the age of 65 show symptoms of Alzheimer's dementia.[3] Among the population over 80, the percentage is much higher: 50% show symptoms of dementia. The average duration of the disease is from 8 to 12 years, but cases can range from 3 to 20 years.

Is Alzheimer's a hereditary disease? If one of my parents or siblings has or had dementia, does it mean I will develop it too?

Relatives of people having dementia, especially sons and daughters, ask if they are more likely to be diagnosed with these diseases because they already have a parent with this diagnosis. Many of these sons and daughters do not know at what age Alzheimer's disease usually starts and are afraid it can hit them at any moment.

In the population over 65 around 10% have dementia. If we look at the population with same age, but among those who had or have siblings or parents with dementia, the percentage is around 20%.

---

[3] Alzheimer's Association. (2018). *2018 Alzheimer's Disease Facts and Figures.* (PDF file) P.17. Washington, DC, USA. Retrieved from https://www.alz.org/facts/

7

"Scientists know genes are involved in Alzheimer's. Two categories of genes influence whether a person develops a disease: risk genes and deterministic genes. Alzheimer's genes have been found in both categories....1) Risk genes increase the likelihood of developing a disease, but do not guarantee it will happen... 2) Deterministic genes directly cause a disease, guaranteeing that anyone who inherits one will develop the disorder".[4]

Only from 1% to 5% of patients with Alzheimer's disease have this deterministic gene and in this case early symptoms start around 50 years old, as happens to Julianne Moore, who plays the main character in the movie "Still Alice", 2014.

In all the other cases there is a genetic risk factor (associated to the gene ApoE 3,4,5), which increases the risk of developing the disease, but does not necessarily trigger the disease.

What are the early typical symptoms?

- Memory loss that disrupts daily life
- Challenges in planning or solving problems
- Difficulty completing familiar tasks at home, at work or at leisure
- Confusion about time or place
- Trouble understanding visual images and spatial relationships
- New problems with words in speaking or writing
- Misplacing things and losing the ability to retrace steps
- Decreased or poor judgment

---

[4] Alzheimer's Association. (2018). Risk factors. Retrieved from https://alz.org/alzheimers_disease_causes_risk_factors.asp

8

- Withdrawal from work or social activities
- Changes in mood and personality

When delirium, hallucinations, and delusions appear, it could mean the patient is getting into the middle stage.

A person diagnosed with Alzheimer's will not necessarily develop all symptoms. It is rare to meet two persons with dementia who look the same. Unless a person has a very risky invasive procedure, undertaken for other reasons than getting a dementia diagnosis, Alzheimer's can be diagnosed with certainty only by a post mortem cerebral biopsy. Sometimes a person diagnosed with a chronic-degenerative disease causing dementia, gets a new and different diagnosis after some years. Some patients have diagnostic errors. Some of them are "false positives", but others are medical errors. This also happens because decoding symptoms is never easy. Symptoms can seem quite clear one day, less evident the day after.

Is it normal aging or Alzheimer's disease?

Today around 10% of people over the age of 65 show symptoms of dementia and around another 40% have some memory deficits. These deficits are "age-associated memory impairment" and are a normal part of aging. If these memory deficits are not the consequence of an underlying medical condition, they are considered as a part of the normal aging process, but sometimes they can be confused with early symptoms of Alzheimer's disease or another dementia. Symptoms that may indicate dementia are different and are not a part of normal aging. Doctors can help a person to distinguish normal age-related memory deficits from symptoms that may indicate dementia. It is important to know when it makes sense to go to

9

your doctor about memory deficits, but it is equally important to consider that forgetting someone's name does not necessarily mean that you are getting dementia. There are differences between early signals of Alzheimer's disease and memory deficits related to normal aging. For instance, if someone does not remember the content of a phone conversation with her/his sister, which occurred four months ago, this can happen in normal aging. But if someone does not remember the content of what she/he said last night, the lapse could merit a medical visit.

If a person meets a friend whom she/he has not seen for years and she/he does not remember the name, it is fine. But it is another thing if this person meets a cousin and is not able to remember her/his name.

If a person does not find a word during a conversation, it may still be fine. If this person cannot have a normal conversation because she/he does not remember words, it makes sense to go to doctor to get a better understanding of it.

To experience "senior moments" means that our brain is slowing down, and does not mean we need to panic.

Here are some easy ways to compare the signs of Alzheimer's vs. typical age-related changes.[5]

- Poor judgment and decision making vs. making a bad decision once in a while

---

[5]Alzheimer's Association. (2011) *Is it Alzheimer's or just signs of aging?* (PDF file). P.1 Retrieved from
https://www.alz.org/national/documents/aa_brochure_10warnsigns.pdf

- Inability to manage a budget vs. missing a monthly payment
- Losing track of the date or the season vs. forgetting which day it is and remembering later
- Difficulty finding the right words to have a conversion vs. sometimes forgetting which word to use
- Misplacing things and being unable to retrace steps to find them vs. losing things from time to time.

The family caregivers

Politics may keep declaring itself to be strongly committed to developing effective policies to support families caring for dementia sufferers, but family caregivers are still the most important resource for their care and are the crucial figures in their care. Without family caregivers, dementia patients' care would collapse in few days, impacting dramatically the health care system's costs.

"*Eighty-three percent of the help provided to older adults in the United States comes from family members, friends or other unpaid caregivers*".[6]

Over the last 12 years, I have studied and supported people suffering from dementia at home and their family caregivers (both in Italy and in the USA). After 12 years I can say that three main factors make the difference in how family caregivers face such an experience during the years they care for loved ones. I can also say that, regardless of the country where

---

[6]Alzheimer's Association. (2018). *2018 Alzheimer's Disease Facts and Figures*. (PDF file) P.31. Washington, DC, USA. Retrieved from https://www.alz.org/facts/

11

patients live and regardless of the standards of their healthcare systems, the three factors are the same:

1. Family financial resources.

The plan of care provided by Medicare or Medicaid maybe unable to cover the real number of needed hours. The Italian public healthcare system is never able to do it. Family financial resources are required to establish a concrete plan of home care. When all the care is funded by the family, the main family caregivers involuntarily become the organizers. It happens, in NYS as in Italy, that families often hire home workers with little expertise or specific education for dementia patients.

2. Family "emotional" and "loving" resources.

The number of family members available to spend and sacrifice themselves for years for the sake of the loved one is crucial. This tough experience discloses the real values of that family. Not everyone in the world who is suffering from dementia can rely on a sufficient number of family members to support them with dedication and love. Young families are increasingly disrupted. Sometimes they are pressed by financial urgencies, sometimes they do not have time or energy, other times they do not want to help their relatives with Alzheimer's.

3. The meaning of sufferance.

What is the sense of this experience? What meaning is given to this experience of pain and stress by the main family caregiver? During this long way, Faith in God, (whatever one's re-

12

ligion) helps many families and family caregivers to reinterpret the sense of this path, accepting the pain and the disease. Faith aids one not to feed that anger which could be lethal for the family members.

When some of these factors do not work, the fog starts to take over the family. The path is already known and for many families, unfortunately, there is no way out. The families must avoid isolation, because loneliness is killing families no less than Alzheimer's.

A family with a member suffering from Alzheimer's, or other dementia, is a family that tends to isolate itself and have difficulty maintaining the lifestyle it had in the past, whatever this lifestyle was. The family is often isolated, as if in a jail. The patient becomes a phantom and the family looks desperately for some times for a respite from a continuous burden, a psychological and physical weight, lasting seven days a week. Over these years, relatives often disappear and the patient's friends struggle to maintain a human and social relationship with the patient. Family caregivers do not come out unscathed from caring at home for a person suffering from dementia.

Many books written by family caregivers around the world perfectly reveal how the social withdrawal of the family is concurrent with an economic depletion. Around the world, health care systems barely focus on people with dementia and not at all on those taking care of them. Systems ignore how expensive it will be not to take care of family caregivers concurrently with patients. In the meantime, not all families survive, and family caregivers are alone, consuming themselves

13

in a cry of pain that nobody listens to, and which, when heard, remains unanswered.

In the book *The Father Who Did Not Know My Name*, the author, Father James Sheehan, faces the theme of isolation and loneliness in taking care a loved one suffering from Alzheimer's disease, an isolation not sparing even a Catholic priest, "a professional of pain". This isolation does not spare anyone, not even those who should have the tools to make sense of pain and manage it. But despite all this sadness, the book can still bring out a positive message. It seems a paradox, but it is so.

Who are the family caregivers? And how can they be supported?

More than 16 million Americans provide unpaid care for people with Alzheimer's or other dementias. Around two-thirds of family caregivers are women. And 34% are age 65 or older.[7]

According to a 2009 study by the National Academy of Sciences, 62% of family caregivers take care of a parent or father/mother-in-law.

At the beginning of the disease a family caregiver has around 15 hours a week for her/himself; by the final stage, this has shrunk to 4 hours.

"According to the 2014 Alzheimer's Association Women and Alzheimer's Poll, which surveyed both men and women, of those providing care for 21 to more than 60 hours per week, 67 percent were women. Similarly, the 2015 BRFSS (Behav-

---

[7] *Ibid.*

14

ioral Risk Factor Surveillance System) survey found that of all dementia caregivers who spend more than 40 hours per week providing care, 69 percent were women. Two and a half times as many women reported living with the person with dementia full time".[8]

Family caregivers find themselves cast in new roles; the most frequent involve:

- Financial Management
- Cooking, Bathing, Dressing
- Nursing
- Providing Recreational Therapy
- Acting as Home Health Aide
- Acting as Social Worker
- Providing Transportation
- Acting as Lawyer

The effects of caregiving on a family caregiver

The onset and progression of dementia are very stressful for the family caregiver. The "objective stressors" lead the family caregivers to psychological stress and impaired health. These objective stressors can also be personally amplified.

Caring for an Alzheimer's patient can negatively affect the caregiver's employment. Nine percent of the family caregivers who are employed have to quit their jobs and 18% have to reduce their work hours due to care responsibilities. Fifty-seven percent go late to work or leave it early. In these situations family caregivers have to choose between economic security

---

[8] *Ibid.*

15

and caring for their love ones. If you compare these data with those of family caregivers of persons suffering from others diseases, you will realize that the percentages for dementia caregivers are definitely higher.[9]

Fortunately, in New York State, since January 1, 2018, *"New York State's Paid Family Leave provides New Yorkers with job-protected, paid leave to care for a loved one with a serious health condition"*[10], but it is not the same all over the US.

The *"2018 Alzheimer's Disease Facts and Figures"* also reports that between 30% and 40% of family caregivers of people with dementia suffer from depression. Non-caregiver peers of similar ages have a depression rate of only between 5% and 17%.

It seems there is a difference in how men and women experience depression arising from taking care of a loved with dementia. *"Women experience depression at a higher rate than men. Women, primarily wives and daughters, provide the majority of caregiving. In the United States, approximately 12 million women experience clinical depression each year, at approximately twice the rate of men.... A Mental Health America study found that many women do not seek treatment for depression because they are embarrassed or in denial about being depressed. In fact, 41% of women surveyed cited embarrassment or shame as barriers to treatment"*.[11]

---

[9] *Ibid.*
[10] New York State. Programs New York State paid family leaving. Retrieved from https://www.ny.gov/programs/new-york-state-paid-family-leave
[11] Reviewed by Beth MacLeod. (2002, 2008, 2016). *Depression and caregiving.* Family Caregiver Alliance. Retrieved from https://www.caregiver.org/depression-and-caregiving

16

Men also do not like to admit their depression. *"Although male caregivers tend to be more willing than female caregivers to hire outside help for assistance with home care duties, they tend to have fewer friends to confide in or positive activities to engage in outside the home. The mistaken assumption that depressive symptoms are a sign of weakness can make it especially difficult for men to seek help".[12]*

As principal researcher, I started in 2015 in Italy a study of how caregiving impacts the health of family caregivers and patients living at home when they cannot rely on educational support. I also realized a possible correlation between emotional stresses of family caregivers and how well or poorly they take care of patients. My study also tends to investigate a correlation between family caregivers with higher scores on a Depression Scale and greater frequency of patients' admission to the Emergency Room. Some of these visits to the E.R. will become admissions to the hospital, including to the ICU (Intensive Care Unit). Is the inefficiency of the family caregiver the cause of an avoidable admission to hospital for the loved one? Or is the burden of the patient care the cause of the depression in the family caregiver? It is a vicious cycle.

The likelihood of using emergency system's care, like 911 and the E.R., is higher for family caregivers of patients with Alzheimer's or another dementia in comparison with the average. *"In separate studies, hospitalization and emergency department visits were more likely for dementia caregivers who*

---

[12] *Ibid.*

17

helped care for recipients who were depressed, had low functional status or had behavioral disturbances".[13]

"*A broad range of outcome measures has been examined, including cellular and organ-based physiologic measures, global physical and psychiatric health status indicators, and self-reports on health habits. These outcomes have been linked to primary stressors, such as the duration and type of care provided and the functional and cognitive disabilities of the care recipient, as well as to secondary stressors, such as finances and family conflict. As a result of these stressors, the caregiver may experience effects such as psychological distress, impaired health habits, physiologic responses, psychiatric illness, physical illness, and even death... Recently researchers have focused not only on providing care as a cause of distress but also on the caregiver's perception of how much the patient is suffering. Patient suffering is manifested in three related and measurable ways: overt physical signs, including verbal and nonverbal expressions of pain and physical discomfort, such as difficulty breathing; psychological symptoms of distress, such as depression and apathy; and existential or spiritual well-being, reflecting the extent to which religious or philosophical beliefs provide inner harmony, comfort, and strength or, alternatively, lead to despair*".[14]

Family caregivers also have a higher mortality rate than other people of the same age. In the article "A Population at Risk"

---

[13] Alzheimer's Association. (2018). *2018 Alzheimer's Disease Facts and Figures*. (PDF file) P.40. Washington, DC, USA. Retrieved from https://www.alz.org/facts/
[14] Schulz, R., Sherwood, P.R., (2008). Physical and Mental Health Effects of Family Caregiving. American *Journal of Nursing*, 108 (9), 23–27. Retrieved from https://www.ncbi.nlm.nih.gov/pmc/articles/PMC2791523/
doi: 10.1097/01.NAJ.0000336406.45248.4c

published on "Family Caregiver Alliance"[15], some interesting studies about family caregivers have discovered these troubling statistics:

"Caregivers also reported chronic conditions (including heart attack/heart disease, cancer, diabetes and arthritis) at nearly twice the rate of non caregivers (45 vs. 24%).[16]

"Caregivers suffer from increased rates of physical ailments (including acid reflux, headaches, and pain/aching)[17]*, increased tendency to develop serious illness*[18]*, and have high levels of obesity and bodily pain.*[19]

"Studies demonstrate that caregivers have diminished immune response, which leads to frequent infection and increased risk of cancers.[20][21][22] *For example, caregivers have a 23% higher*

---

[15] Reviewed by Moira Fordyce. (2006). *Caregiver health.* Family Caregiver Alliance. Retrieved from https://www.caregiver.org/caregiver-health

[16] Ho, A., Collins, S., Davis, K. & Doty, M. (2005). *A Look at Working-Age Caregivers Roles, Health Concerns, and Need for Support* (Issue Brief). New York, NY: The Commonwealth Fund.

[17] National Alliance for Caregiving & Evercare. (2006). *Evercare® Study of Caregivers in Decline: A Close-up Look at the Health Risks of Caring for a Loved One.* Bethesda, MD: National Alliance for Caregiving and Minnetonka, MN: Evercare.

[18] Shaw, W.S., Patterson, T.L., Semple, S.J., Ho, S., Irwin, M.R., Hauger, R.L. & Grant, I. (1997). Longitudinal analysis of multiple indicators of health decline among spousal caregivers. *Annals of Behavioral Medicine,* 19: 101-109.

[19] Barrow, S. & Harrison, R. (2005). Unsung heroes who put their lives at risk? Informal caring, health, and neighborhood attachment. *Journal of Public Health,* 27(3): 292-297.

[20] Kiecolt-Glaser, J.K., Dura, J.R. & Speicher, C.E., (1991). Spousal caregivers of dementia victims: Longitudinal changes in immunity and health. *Psychosomatic Medicine,* 53(4):345-362.

[21] Kiecolt-Glaser, J., Glaser, R., Gravenstein, S., Malarkey, W.B. & Sheridan, J.,(1996). *Chronic stress alters the immune response to influenza virus vaccine in older adults.* Proceedings of the National Academy of Sciences of the United States of America, 93: 3043-3047.

19

level of stress hormones and a 15% lower level of antibody responses.[23] Caregivers also suffer from slower wound healing.[24]

"The physical stress of caregiving can affect the physical health of the caregiver, especially when providing care for someone who cannot transfer him/herself out of bed, walk or bathe without assistance. Ten percent of primary caregivers report that they are physically strained"[25].

The burden of taking care impacts not only the health of the patient and family caregivers, but also impacts relationships among relatives, and families can fall apart under the strain of arguments.

The situation is difficult also when a son or daughter lives far from the city where another sibling is taking care of their parent. The distant siblings would like to help, and then they start to talk to the one who is taking care in order to help. Many times taking care of a patient at home makes a family caregiver feel overwhelmed, stressed and judged.

Associations for patients can help to support family members coping with this tough disease, providing a lot of useful programs for them as well.

---

[22] Glaser, R. & Kiecolt-Glaser, J.K. (1997). Chronic stress modulates the virus-specific immune response to latent herpes simplex virus Type 1. *Annals of Behavioral Medicine*, 19: 78-82

[23] Vitaliano, P., Zhang, J. & Scanlan, J. (2003). Is caregiving hazardous to one's physical health? A meta-analysis. *Psychological Bulletin*, 129(6): 946-972.

[24] Kiecolt-Glaser, J.K., Marucha, P.T., Malarkey, W.B., Mercado, A.M. & Glaser, R. (1996) Slowing of wound healing by psychological stress. *Lancet*, 346(8984): 1194-1196.

[25] Center on Aging Society. (2005). *How Do Family Caregivers Fare? A Closer Look at Their Experiences.* (Data Profile, Number 3). Washington, DC: Georgetown University.

Alzheimer's Association in the document "*2018 Alzheimer's Disease Facts and Figures*"[26] reports that there are several useful types of Family Caregiver Interventions:

" *Case management. Provides assessment, information, planning, referral, care coordination and/or advocacy for family caregivers.*

"*Psycho-educational approaches. Include a structured program that provides information about the disease, resources and services, and about how to expand skills to effectively respond to symptoms of the disease (that is, cognitive impairment, behavioral symptoms and care-related needs). Include lectures, discussions and written materials and are led by professionals with specialized training.*

"*Counseling. Aims to resolve pre-existing personal problems that complicate caregiving to reduce conflicts between caregivers and care recipients and/or improve family functioning.*

"*Support groups. Are less structured than psycho-educational or psychotherapeutic interventions. Support groups provide caregivers the opportunity to share personal feelings and concerns to overcome feelings of social isolation.*

"*Respite. Provides planned, temporary relief for the caregiver through the provision of substitute care; examples include adult day services and in-home or institutional respite for a certain number of weekly hours.*

---

[26] Alzheimer's Association. (2018). *2018 Alzheimer's Disease Facts and Figures*. (PDF file) P.40. Washington, DC, USA. Retrieved from https://www.alz.org/facts/

"Psychotherapeutic approaches. Involve the establishment of a therapeutic relationship between the caregiver and a professional therapist (for example, cognitive-behavioral therapy for caregivers to focus on identifying and modifying beliefs related to emotional distress, developing new behaviors to deal with caregiving demands, and fostering activities that can promote caregiver well-being).

"Multicomponent approaches. Are characterized by intensive support strategies that combine multiple forms of interventions, such as education, support and respite into a single, long-term service (often provided for 12 months or more)".

Some scientists studied how nursing home admission for family caregivers of people with dementia could be delayed with psycho-educational approaches. These interventions aimed at reducing the caregivers' burden and depression.[27]

Despite scientific evidences about family caregiver interventions, *"a 2016 study of the Older Americans Act's National Family Caregiver Support Program found that over half (52%) of Area Agencies on Aging did not offer evidence-based family caregiver interventions"*[28].

Some interventions based on cognitive and behavioral therapies achieved a decrease in the number of family caregivers with depression and improved their psychological well-being. *"Subjective strain is the appraisal of burden by the caregiver, including their evaluation of the physical and emotional im-*

---

[27] Brodaty, H., Donkin, M. (2009). Family caregivers of people with dementia. *Dialogues in Clinical neuroscience.* Jun 11(2): 217–228. Retrieved from https://www.ncbi.nlm.nih.gov/pmc/articles/PMC3181916/ PMID: 19585957

[28] Alzheimer's Association. (2018). *2018 Alzheimer's Disease Facts and Figures.* (PDF file) P.41. Washington, DC, USA. Retrieved from https://www.alz.org/facts/

pact, their psychological state, and resources. Subjective strain is only loosely correlated with objective burden. Caregivers generally report experiencing some form of strain"[29].

Dementia Diary

When a family has collapsed under the burden and the stress over the years, or when a family caregiver is diagnosed with a disease triggered by years of burden, it may be too late for recovery. I developed the educational program, called *Dementia Diary*. It provides specific tips for family caregivers suggesting how they may fight loss of dignity of the patients and notice and respond to safety red flags. And *Dementia Diary* can also support family caregivers s psychologically.

It is a tool to educate not only family caregivers but also home workers in order to reduce stress of the family caregivers, to preserve safety and dignity of the patient. The tool, called *Dementia Diary*, was developed and copyrighted in 2008. It involves a one-to-one meeting between the family caregiver and a trained professional to educate her/him to handle at-home events with a patient with Alzheimer's or another dementia.

Dementia Diary addresses the problems of family caregivers who need customized information and suggestions to handle, solve or simply understand emerging new problems. Different home settings, socio-economic contexts, and stages of the disease require different type of tips. This tool is also a great

---

[29] *Ibid.*

23

way to educate nurses, social workers and any type of home workers.

Dementia Diary catalogs hundreds of events occurring at home in the daily life of the patient, the family caregiver or both. The events are taken from both a worldwide scientific literature and my personal observations during my home care visits. For every event there is at least one tip. After a screening of hundreds of events, covering all the clinical characteristics from the beginning to the final stage, the family caregiver will receive a catalogue of information that can be described as hyper-personalized tips from a great number of suggestions, also gathered over many years, both from my study of international literature and from my observation of patients.

When I used *Dementia Diary*, I could see how family caregivers learned information needed to acquire relevant skills, to develop right behaviors, especially about safety and dignity of the loved one, and to handle their own emotions.

This list is supplemented by a monthly phone call that aims at verifying whether the family caregiver or the worker is following the recommendations and if additional information is needed.

Calling the family caregiver also aims at encouraging her/him to learn better the recommendations tailored to the patient's life.

The new concept is the management of the relationship at home, between family caregiver (or home worker) and patient with Alzheimer's disease or other dementia, including practical tips to follow non-pharmacological interventions. *Demen-*

24

tia Diary can impact the family caregivers' mood and consequently be a great help in preventing family caregivers from falling into depression. It could also be an effective way to limit the number of avoidable hospitalizations, even if appropriate, for both the patient and the family caregiver.

II

HEALTHY LIFESTYLES

Can healthy lifestyles prevent dementia, delay its onset or slow its progress?

There is no cure for most neurodegenerative diseases showing dementia symptoms, and doctors can only prescribe symptomatic drugs, easing some symptoms. But their effect is only temporary.

Despite Alzheimer's incurability, there is good news: neuroprotection. *Neuroprotective* means to be able to slow down pathological or physiological loss of nerve cells in the brain. Some healthy lifestyles can be crucial for our brain's health. They include specific activities, considered neuroprotective. Some of these neuroprotective activities are also able to boost the neuroplasticity of the brain.

The adult brain can even generate new nerve cells: this is called *neuroplasticity*. A neuroscientist, Jonas Frisen from Karolinska Institutet (Sweden), says that we produce around 700 new neurons a day in the hippocampus. This ability to produce new neurons slows down over the years.

Neuroplasticity "*is the brain's ability to reorganize itself by forming new neural connections throughout life. Neuroplastic-*

ity allows the neurons (nerve cells) in the brain to compensate for injury and disease and to adjust their activities in response to new situations or to changes in their environment"[30].

Based on scientific studies, the six following neuroprotective activities are considered very effective to slow down the physiological and pathological loss of neurons and sometimes partially to restore them, and consequently to reduce risk for developing dementia symptoms.

1. Doing Physical Exercise. Do at least 40/45 minutes' aerobic activity daily, such as a brisk walk. New connections and nerve cells are born, neuro-inflammation decreases and amyloid plaques are dissolved.

2. Having a Healthy Diet. Follow the Mediterranean diet for instance (see the Chapter Three of this book). You must also try to avoid bad habits like drinking too much alcohol.

3. Staying Socially Engaged. Avoid loneliness. It does not mean necessarily going to dances or to parties every day, but loneliness "kills" people. Having four/five friends, talking or meeting some of them daily is essential to avoid social isolation. Interacting with children or grandchildren is effective, too. An intense social life, rich in relationship, can lower the risk of developing dementia symptoms. To have the desired protective effect, the relationship must:

- involve interacting with others actually (not virtually), and

---

[30] Medical definition of Neuroplasticity. (2017).
Retrieved from https://www.medicinenet.com/script/main/art.asp?articlekey=40362

27

- stimulate our intellect (an interaction full of meaning for the mind).

4. Learning New Things. For instance, learning to speak a new language or play a music instrument. This is different and better than activities like puzzles or computer games. These are effective in keeping the brain trained, but they retrieve memories already there in the brain. Learning new things boosts new neurons' developing and supports the brain's plasticity. It is important because in this way new synapses are created in the brain, allowing new connections between nerve cells. The hippocampus must work properly to learn new things, and it is the area of the brain most affected by Alzheimer.

5. Reducing Emotional Stresses. Do meditation or take a yoga class. You can learn to practice mindful breathing techniques. You can also protect your brain from harmful neurochemicals like cortisol, by avoiding all stressful situations. Catholic contemplative prayer, as described in *The Catechism*, is similar to the meditation we are talking about. If you are a believer in God, you will be able to practice contemplative prayer; if not, you could learn meditation methods and breathing techniques.

6. Getting Seven/Eight Hours of Sleep. Our brains are systems, needing a nightly back up. R. Tanzi[31] says, *"it is during the deepest stage of sleep (delta or slow-wave) following dreams (REM sleep) that the brain clears itself of debris like*

---

[31] Rudolph Tanzi is the Joseph P. and Rose F. Kennedy Professor of Neurology at Harvard University, and Director of the Genetics and Aging Research Unit at Massachusetts General Hospital

amyloid plaques. This is also when short-term memories are consolidated into long-term memories"[32].

The abnormal accumulation of the proteins, beta-amyloid and tau, seems to start from ten to twenty years before early dementia symptoms. Scientists have not yet found a pharmacological intervention to stop or slow down abnormal accumulation of these substances. Neither have they found a cure.

So there are social and personal habits, which are neuroprotective, able to reduce the risk of developing dementia or to delay the onset of early symptoms or to slow down the progression of the symptoms. Following these neuroprotective activities with great regularity means to be part of the low-risk group for developing dementia rather the high-risk group.

Promoting these non-pharmacological interventions in the communities could be as important for 45-year-olds as for the elderly. And among the elderly, the interventions benefit both those with dementia and those with memory deficits normally related to aging. According to scientific studies and guidelines, DNA alone does not determine if we will get Alzheimer's, except for that 1%-5% of patients with Alzheimer's disease having deterministic genes. And following these lifestyles in daily life helps to accomplish important goals for brain health in different categories of people.

- *Among people suffering from dementia*, it could slow down the progression of symptoms.
- *For persons over 60 without dementia*, it could delay or prevent the possible onset of symptoms or the pos-

---

[32] Chopra D.,Tanzi R., (2018) *The Healing self.* Harmony books, New York, USA.

29

sible onset of memory and cognitive deficits (those considered "age-associated memory impairment").

- *For persons in their 40s and 50s*, it may delay or prevent the possible future onset of memory and cognitive deficits.

There is something we cannot neglect to cite here. In the article "Dementia prevention, intervention, and care", published in July 2017, in the British medical journal *Lancet*, scientists say that nine factors might have the potential to delay or prevent one third (35%) of dementia cases. They are *"getting an education (staying in school until over the age of fifteen); reducing high blood pressure, obesity and diabetes; avoiding or treating hearing loss in mid-life; not smoking; getting physical exercise; and reducing depression and social isolation later in life"*[33]. With these studies doctors push persons to focus on their lifestyle twenty or thirty years before the first symptoms; it is called the "incremental medicine".

---

[33] Livingston G, Sommerlad A, Orgeta V, Costafreda S G, Huntley J, Ames D, Ballard C, Banerjee S, Burns A, Cohen-Mansfield J, Cooper C, Fox N, Gitlin L N, Howard R, Kales H C, Larson E B, Ritchie K, Rockwood K, Sampson E L, Samus Q, Schneider L S, Selbæk G, Teri L, Mukadam N (2017). Dementia prevention, intervention, and care. *The Lancet*. Vol. 390, No. 10113
Retrieved from https://www.ncbi.nlm.nih.gov/pubmed/28735855
DOI:10.1016/S0140-6736(17)31363-6

30

Quality indicators and standards in healthy lifestyles

In order to define quality standards, we need first to identify quality indicators. An indicator expresses a specific phenomenon in quantitative terms; it is a "quantitative definition". We want to measure how well our brain's health is preserved or improved through a particular lifestyle.

For this purpose, I identify two indicators sets. One is about social life and the other concerns the brain's health. The first measures how much the healthy lifestyles are really implemented in the daily life. The second investigates the health impact that this lifestyle has on the brain. We want to know how healthy lifestyles impact the daily life both: of people suffering from dementia, slowing down the progression of their symptoms; and of people over 60 years old, delaying the onset of early dementia symptoms or normal memory deficits.

The first indicators (social life) are of particular interest to ordinary people willing to adopt a new lifestyle, and do it well. Ordinary people and experts in the field would be interested in and encouraged by both types of indicators.

We need to know when can we say a person is correctly following a specific lifestyle healthy for the brain. What are the requisite actions? Who defines what they are? For how long must a person comply with the "new rules" to be said to have a new, lasting lifestyle?

Having determined the answers to these questions, and based on that time frame, we can measure how well a person is following this lifestyle.

When TV popularizes a study, as when CNN announced that "those who say they followed the diet religiously had a 53% lower chance of getting Alzheimer's, while those who followed it moderately lowered their risk by about 35%", what does it mean? What do non-experts mean by the concepts of "religious" and "moderate"? The terms "religious" and "moderate" lack of scientific precision, and this annuls the seeming exactitude of the percentages.

Every lifestyle healthy for the brain requires a different amount of time to be considered part of one's life and takes a different amount of time to have an impact on the brain's health, for example: the time required for results to show is much longer for following a diet than for doing physical exercise. Some health indicators can be measured only over a span of years. Others immediately after a person has finished an activity. For instance how mood changes after 45 minutes of brisk walking is different from how a healthy meal could impact your brain.

In order to acquire and keep lifelong habits, it is important to introduce changes gradually. Studies show that making little changes over time is more effective than making sudden, drastic change. For instance, to start a new healthy diet you could begin by gradually eliminating junk food and increasing your intake of fruit and vegetables.

The development of measures for home health is in the early stages, but we already have some Home Health Quality Measures for Consumers. Institute of Medicine categorized The Six Domains of Health Care Quality, where only some of them are for home health care.

I do not think we can ask patients to follow new healthy lifestyles for the brain without measuring whether these lifestyles affect at least some of the indicators in the list below. In fact some of them could be easily related to some dementia symptoms. So, even if these patients do not have home health care provided by an agency, it would make sense to monitor some of these indicators. This will help us to understand how healthy lifestyles can be considered effective to slow down the progression of clinical symptoms. Therefore, it would make sense also to measure the effectiveness of the social programs provided at Saint Thomas More Church, New York, for patients with dementia, using some of these indicators, especially when they do not have home health care provided by an agency.

Among the indicators categorized in The Six Domains of Health Care Quality, I found these to be most appropriate.

"Patient Safety Measures:

- *Percentage of patients needing emergent care for wound infections or deteriorating wound status.*

- *Percentage of patients who require emergent care from a hospital, doctor, or outpatient department/clinic for any type of emergency.*

Effectiveness Measures:

- *Percentage of patients showing improvement in, for example,*
  - *Ambulation/locomotion.*
  - *Bathing.*
  - *Management of oral medications.*
  - *Status of surgical wounds.*
  - *Urinary incontinence"[34].*

We can use other indicators to understand where healthy lifestyles should impact in the life of people with dementia.

Until recently, Medicare used the following set of indicators when comparing home care agencies which they reimbursed.

- Percentage of patients who do not get worse in the ability to ambulate.
- Percentage of patients who do not get worse when they enter and leave their bed.
- Percentage of patients who do not increase the number of incontinence episodes.
- Percentage of patients who do not get worse in taking a bath.
- Percentage of patients who improve the correct intake of drugs (per month).
- Percentage of patients who do not have a greater number of episodes of dyspnea.

---

[34] Examples of Home Health Quality Measures for consumers. Agency for Healthcare Research and Quality.
Retrieved from https://www.ahrq.gov/professionals/quality-patient-safety/talkingquality/create/longtermcare/homehealthcare/examples.html

- Percentage of patients who stay home after home health care.
- Percentage of patients who were hospitalized.
- Percentage of patients who need an urgent and unplanned medical assistance.

The above set of indicators seems to me still usable today. And, of course, a set of indicators for patient safety can also be used. They will help us to understand and measure the magnitude of the impact of a lifestyle or a program on the patient's safety.

Safety indicators

- Percentage of patients fallen
- Percentage of patients who got lost, out of home
- Percentage of patients near to choking
- Percentage of patients poisoned by drugs or chemical substances
- Percentage of patients with cuts
- Percentage of patients burned

Certainly, I am not here asserting that there is a unique cause-effect nexus. If patient safety is improved or progression of symptoms slowed down, this does not mean that they happened solely due attending the program or following the lifestyle.

Can people with dementia live normally in their community? Observation at Saint Thomas More Church, NY

I experienced at Saint Thomas More Church that people with dementia could live normally in their community.

What can a family caregiver do to assure good health care for a dementia patient living at home? Are drugs alone sufficient? Is there anything else we can do for them?

When in 2010 I founded GP Dementia Services NY, this foundation had the purpose of:

- providing support group services, which entails educating and providing information to persons suffering from dementia and to families, primarily low-income families, which have members suffering from dementia; and
- reducing depression, anxiety and other forms of emotional distress among family members who take care of persons suffering from dementia.

I began, in January 2017, to organize some new programs at Saint Thomas More Church in New York. The participants were limited to people suffering from dementia and their families. All the programs were based on neuroprotective activities.

By May 2017, although the purposes written in 2010 were still the same, my thoughts on how to accomplish them were changing. Something more was needed for the programs. Due to my reading of recent scientific studies, I realized that these programs could be effective not only for people suffering from dementia (in order to slow down the progression of the symptoms) but also for the elderly without cognitive impairment (in order to delay a possible onset of dementia or some memory and cognitive deficits which are part of normal aging in 40% of people over 65 years old).

So in May 2017 I changed the policy to extend all programs to all seniors, even those without any pathological cognitive impairment. So individuals from both groups started to benefit form these programs.

Why did I understand we needed this change in taking care people suffering from dementia? It had become clear to me how important it was to provide more social, non-pharmacological interventions and not only pharmacological interventions.

Recent scientific literature indicates that non-pharmacological therapies for patients can support patients with dementia; they help to slow down the symptoms of disease. They also improve quality of life, preserve dignity and increase safety. The therapies below are the most important and most frequently used by caregivers.

Some of them are called "Standard therapies", such as Behavioral therapy, Reality orientation, Validation therapy, and Reminiscence therapy.

Others, termed "Alternative therapies", include Art therapy, Music therapy, Activity therapy, Complementary therapy, Aromatherapy, Bright-light therapy, Multisensory approaches.

Another group, known as "Brief psychotherapies", contains Cognitive-behavioral therapy and Interpersonal therapy.

Most of these therapies must be provided by professionals. They are usually provided at Adult Day Health Care Centers with Special Alzheimer's Units – much less often by home-workers. It is also true that:

- Few who suffer from dementia attend an Adult Day Health Care Center.
- Providing these therapies at home, where most of the patients live, is very expensive and difficult.

If we know these therapies better, we will able to understand how they can apply to ordinary moments of daily life of persons suffering from dementia. The goal of the programs of the foundation at Saint Thomas More Church is to turn the essentials of these therapies into healthy daily lifestyle.

In this way the programs' goals were automatically extended from "supporting families and people affected with dementia" to "preventing, postponing or slowing down all the pathological and physiological cognitive and memory decline in people over 60 years old".

In these new programs, the only two requirements for attendance were 1) to be over 60 years old and 2) to undergo a Mini Mental Status Examination (MMSE).[35]

---

[35] *Folstein MF, Folstein SE, McHugh PR, (1975) Mini-mental state: a practical method for grading the cognitive state of patients for the clinician.* Journal of psychiatric research. 12(3):189-98. Retrieved from https://www.ncbi.nlm.nih.gov/pubmed/1202204 PMID: 1202204

Thanks to this change we did more, and better. In fact, under the earlier program, only few people with dementia participated, and they found companionship only with few other persons also suffering from dementia. The new programs allow for inclusion rather than segregation. The step forward was huge.

The change had great consequences. More people attended our programs, and, by taking the MMSE, around 20% of the new participants learned that their scores fell within the dementia range. It was good for those people to get the chance to know it, so that if they wished, they could follow up with a visit to a doctor.

The new social model of the programs gives more because seniors with and without dementia mix together. For people over 60 years without dementia, seeing people with dementia having difficulties, are moved to help them. Elderly people feel good serving others and feeling useful to the others. People over 60 years without dementia are also able to appreciate the simple activities they are still able to perform: walking by themselves, remembering, and other simple things of daily life.

Since September 2017, the programs at Saint Thomas More have burgeoned to five: one to promote each of the six most effective neuroprotective activities, except sleeping at least 7-8 hours.

1. "Physical Activity", with Flamenco class, Latin-American dancing class, and Yoga Class.

2. "Healthy Diet", with "Cooking demonstration" of the Mediterranean diet's dishes. Famous chefs were invited to do the demonstration.
3. "Learning New Things", with three different classes: "Italian Language", "Italian Movies" and Computer and smartphone knowledge".
4. "Socializing", with the Art Buddy Program.
5. "Relieve Your Stress", with a Meditation class.

For every senior I wanted to measure how many times he/she attended the class during the five months' program. Furthermore I wanted to measure the following indicators both at the beginning of the program and after five months from the beginning.

Doing physical activities:
Goal: every person does at least 45 minutes of physical activity a day five days a week.

1. Number of persons doing at least 45 minutes of physical activities five times for week.
2. Number of persons doing at least 45 minutes of physical activities once a week.
3. Number of persons who increased number of days a week when they do at least 45 minutes of physical activities.

Following healthy diet
Goal: every person follows at least seven out of eleven recommendations about healthy diet (see the questionnaire at page 67).

40

1. Number of persons following all eleven healthy recommendations about diet.
2. Number of persons following at least five out of eleven healthy recommendations about diet.
3. Number of persons who increased number of healthy recommendations about diet followed.

Socializing
Goal: every person can talk by phone and/or meet five persons weekly

1. Number of persons having five persons with whom meeting or talking by phone weekly.
2. Number of persons having a person with whom meeting or talking by phone weekly.
3. Number of persons who increased number of persons with whom meeting or talking by phone weekly.

Releasing stress
Goal: every person does at least twenty minutes of mediation a day.

1. Number of persons doing at least twenty minutes of meditation a day.
2. Number of persons doing at least twenty minutes of meditation once a week.
3. Number of persons who increased number of days a week when they do at least twenty minutes of meditation.

Learning new language
Goal: every person learns at least 50 new words in five months

1. Number of persons learning at least 50 new words (two new words a week).
2. Number of persons watching a movie once a month (with English subtitles).
3. Number of persons speaking with someone who is a native speaker of the new language at least once a week.

All the programs were free of charge. They were open to anyone over 60. People suffering from dementia needed to attend programs accompanied by their own caregiver.

We also provided "Support for family caregivers" with two programs: the first involved a one-to-one meeting with me, based on the *Dementia Diary* and follow up calls, and the second provided companionship to people with dementia attending our programs, staffed by volunteers. And the second was only tested.

At Saint Thomas More Church these years, we also organized the following conferences: "Faith, Alzheimer, and parishes", "Neuroprotective activities: adults, patients with dementia and family caregivers", "Dementia: the dignity of the patient and the faith of the family caregiver", "Safety and injury prevention", "Alzheimer's: an opportunity to love", and "Alzheimer's disease: ethics and support for family caregivers".

The purpose of all these programs is definitely also to promote the concept that a person suffering from dementia could live normally with the community, if properly supported. Some-

42

times safety problems become almost an opportunity to prefer a Nursing home or to confine the patient at home, other times there is no choice and Nursing home is the only one. But in both cases we know that some things can make dementia worse, and even hasten its progress. For instance giving patients many drugs or leaving them in an environment without stimulus contributes to negating their personalities and lessen self-esteem.

If it is easy to configure a portrait of a family caregivers of patients with dementia, and, consequently, to organize and provide supports, it is much more complicated to identify the typical dementia patient. Each patient with dementia is unique. Consequently, every plan of social activities for him/her has to be hyper-personalized. This uniqueness of plan requires skills, knowledge and time that not all home care workers and professionals are able to provide. If, then, this list of social activities has to be intuited and organized by the family members, the patient will likely not receive what it would take to live better.

About this approach I agree with Kate Irving,[36] an Irish social worker and expert in dementia. I agree with her when she says that personality, biography and the psychology of patient are as crucial as neurological impairment and physical health. She also says too many drugs and not assuring a stimulating place to live make the patient worse for sure. I think that the last two things also harm the safety and dignity of these persons. And when you do not assure the patient a stimulating place and you treat the disease only by giving medications, you are *de facto*

---

[36] Tedx Talks. (2015, May 22). The Four Myths of Dementia, Kate Irving, TEDxDCU. (Video file).
Retrieved from https://www.youtube.com/watch?v=8a9AguRGmbE

ignoring the personality, biography and the psychology of the patient.

I have always thought of Alzheimer's as not only a diagnosis of a single person, but also a sentence on a family, who will have to cope with this disease daily, and for years. The relatives experience how the personality, biography and the psychology of their own loved ones are destroyed. And the patients lose themselves. In order to help future doctors to not overlook this context, I organized in Italy a program where the first-year medical students, after being trained, spend one hour a week with an Alzheimer's patient for three months.

Irving shows the uniqueness of an Alzheimer's patient; talking about the patient, she says the three criteria necessary to make any diagnosis are

1) etiological validity
2) phenomenological validity
3) prognostic validity.

She goes on to explain why they would not be entirely met by Alzheimer's diagnoses. As for etiological validity, she points out that there are many diseases that can prove these symptoms. Some scientists count 50, others count as many as 200. Diagnostic certainty for Alzheimer's is post-mortem, almost always.

Regarding phenomenological validity, or in the symptoms that the patient shows, we know well how each patient with dementia shows different symptoms both in the first stage, in the intermediate stage and even in the final one.

This is why, when family caregivers are given a sheet with all the symptoms of dementia during the initial support meeting, the professional always reminds them that their loved ones will not exhibit all the listed symptoms. This reminder is both true and reassuring.

For prognostic validity, the diagnosing physician should be able to offer a reliable projection of life expectancy and a trajectory of symptom progression. Neither can be predicted with any confidence and may differ widely in any two patients. Firstly, because an Alzheimer's patient's death may easily be caused by other diseases or by dementia-related factors which are not, themselves, symptoms of dementia. For example, pneumonia that was caused by food getting into the lungs, due to poor ability to swallow (symptom of dementia), can lead to death, particularly in an elderly person. Or a fall that caused a hip fracture in a person over 80 years could lead to post-operative complications that result in death. The fall may have happened because the patient, with recent episodes of slight incontinence, run quickly at night to reach the bathroom. The patient may also fall because the brain's ability to maintain balance was compromised by dementia, so the patient's fall was due solely to dementia.

III

THE MEDITERRANEAN DIET

Background of the Mediterranean diet

Some decades ago, the Mediterranean diet was known only to a very small scientific community. It was a diet coming from a mix of the traditional eating habits in certain areas around the Mediterranean Sea, primarily Spain, South Italy and, above all, Greece.

Not all countries bordering on the Mediterranean Sea were involved with the real Mediterranean diet. For instance diets of some of Mediterranean countries do not include wine and olive oil, which are essential to the Mediterranean diet. Only Spain, South Italy and Greece, out of the 21 countries surrounding the Mediterranean Sea, as observed during the Sixties, are strictly considered to represent the Mediterranean diet. One region is regarded as the epicenter of the Mediterranean diet: Crete, the largest of the Greek isles.

Today, the Mediterranean diet is less followed in the Mediterranean, even in the three regions where it was widespread in the Sixties. Currently, people in these countries eat much red meat and processed and prepackaged food. Concomitantly, the rate of childhood obesity is very high.

Truly, seventy years ago nobody knew what the Mediterranean diet was and in the U.S. some people looked down upon a diet with olive oil and much garlic. It was considered more a part of ethnic food, and not considered a real "diet". The first study about it was done in 1948 by an American physiologist Dr. A. Keys of Rockefeller University, New York. He was studying the possible link between poverty and diet in Crete. Some years later Keys found that men and women from Crete had no coronary disease: this was 1961 and the Greeks had the highest average life expectancy in the world. Their diet, based on unsaturated fat and high in vegetable oils, was observed both in Greece and in Southern Italy during the 1960s.

In 2009, a study by the Harvard Medical School, the World Health Organization and a nonprofit organization "Oldways Preservation and Exchange Trust" produced the famous Mediterranean Diet Food Pyramid. Of course, the Pyramid was based on this diet and they defined the Mediterranean diet as the diet of Crete, the rest of Greek and southern Italy in 1960.

What do you eat with the Mediterranean diet?

Based on a study by Courtney Davis et al. *"Definition of the Mediterranean Diet: A Literature Review"*, *"general descriptions of the Mediterranean Diet are similar amongst publications, emphasizing the same key components. The definitions include guidelines for high intake of extra virgin (cold pressed) olive oil, vegetables including leafy green vegetables, fruits, cereals, nuts and pulses/legumes, moderate intakes of fish and other meat, dairy products and red wine, and low intakes of eggs and sweets. Each description provides an indica-*

47

tion of the frequency these foods should be consumed, for example often, daily, biweekly and the amounts in the diet, described using subjective terms such as abundance, high, moderate, low, some, and vast. Most lack specific suggestions for numbers of servings or serving size, and do not specify amounts of additives to the diet, such as sauces, condiments, tea, coffee, salt, sugar, or honey. Some definitions specify that cereals should be mostly wholegrain"[37].

The Role of the Mediterranean Diet in the Brain and Neurodegenerative Disease, published in 2017, presents a very similar analysis of the groups of foods.[38]

The Mediterranean Diet Pyramid (1993, updated in 2009) of the Oldways Preservation and Exchange Trust recommends eating red meat no more than once a month, to reduce the intake of saturated fats. One study by Mayo Clinic researchers suggests that the high ratio of unsaturated to saturated fats may play a significant part in the Mediterranean diet's benefits to cognitive health.[39]

What is the recommended quantity of food for every serving? How many servings of each food group are recommended? The diet pyramid helps us to understand both.

---

[37] Davis, C. Bryan, J. Hodgson, J. and Murphy, K. (2015). Definition of the Mediterranean Diet: A Literature Review. *Nutrients.* 5;7(11):9139-53. Retrieved from https://www.ncbi.nlm.nih.gov/pubmed/26556369 doi: 10.3390/nu7115459.

[38] Farooqui T, Farooqui A, *Role of the Mediterranean Diet in the Brain and Neurodegenerative Diseases*, Academic Press, San Diego, California, 2017.

[39] Roberts RO, Geda YE, Cerhan JR, Knopman DS, Cha RH, Christianson TJ, Pankratz VS, Ivnik RJ, Boeve BF, O'Connor HM, Petersen RC. (2010). Vegetables, unsaturated fats, moderate alcohol intake, and mild cognitive impairment. *Dementia and geriatric cognitive disorders.* Retrieved from https://www.ncbi.nlm.nih.gov/pmc/articles/PMC2889256/doi: 10.1159/000305099

Three most important pyramids are:

- Oldways Preservation and Exchange Trust (1993, updated in 2009);
- Greek Dietary guidelines (1999);
- Mediterranean Diet Foundation (MDF) (2010).

The three pyramids show the same thirteen food groups

1. Olive oil
2. Vegetables
3. Fruits
4. Breads and cereals
5. Legumes
6. Nuts
7. Fish or Seafood
8. Eggs
9. Poultry
10. Red meat
11. Sweets
12. Red wine
13. Dairy

An interesting article by Courtney Davis et al. presents a table in which 14 studies (from 1990 to 2006) of the Mediterranean diet are reviewed. Differently to what is indicated in the food groups shown in the three pyramids mentioned above, some of the Mediterranean diet variations Davis reviews do not include red wine and sweets as additional food groups.

There were some inconsistencies in classification of food groups between the different studies. For instance some combined fruits and nuts while other separated them, which could be worthwhile, as nuts appear to have an independent role in health.[40]

The three pyramids differ about number of servings per day or meal, or frequency per month or week. Here are the serving sizes, expressed in grams, set forth in Courtney Davis et al.

Food group	Grams	Ounces
Bread	25	0.88
Potato	100	3.52
Cooked pasta	50/60	1.76/2.12
Vegetables	100	3.52
Apple	80	2.82
Banana	60	2.12
Orange	100	3.52
Melon	200	7.05
Grapes	30	1.06
Milk or yogurt	1 cup	1 cup
One egg	-	-
Meat	60	2.12
Cooked dry beans	100	3.52

[40] Souza R.G., Gomes A.C., Naves M.M., Mota J.F. (2015). Nuts and legume seeds for cardiovascular risk reduction: Scientific evidence and mechanisms of action. *Nutrition reviews.* 73(6):335-47. Retrieved from https://www.ncbi.nlm.nih.gov/pubmed/26011909 doi: 10.1093/nutrit/nuu008.

"The three pyramids are similar, but they differ in their recommendations for vegetables and fruits, nuts and legumes, fish/seafood and poultry. Recommendations for legume intake range from every meal to at least twice a week. The [Mediterranean Diet Foundation] suggests daily nuts, while the Greek guidelines are less specific and recommend fewer servings"[41].

The study by Courtney Davis et al. correctly takes into consideration differences based on gender and age: we do not intend to conduct a scientific debate on these data, but to help the reader to acquire a general idea about how much, on average, in grams per day we should eat from every group.

---

[41] Davis C, Bryan J, Hodgson J and Murphy K. (2015). Definition of the Mediterranean Diet: A Literature Review. *Nutrients.* 5;7(11):9139-53. Retrieved from https://www.ncbi.nlm.nih.gov/pubmed/26556369 doi: 10.3390/nu7115459.

Food group	Grams	Ounces
Bread	298.6	10.53
All Cereals	305.8	10.79
Legumes	35.6	1.26
Potato	125.8	4.4
All Vegetables including potatoes	374.9	13.22
Fruits/ Nuts	268.7	9.48
Meat/Meat Products (includes unprocessed and processed red meat, white meat and deli meats)	105.1	3.71
Cheese	21.9	0.77
All Dairy (includes cheese, milk and milk products, and yogurt)	213.6	7,53
Eggs	23	0.81
Olive Oil	44	1.56
Fish (oily fish, non oily fish and shellfish)	50.5	1.78

Online it is possible to find more than one organization, profit or non-profit, providing printable shopping lists of the most common ingredient used to prepare the Mediterranean diet meals.

The Oldways Foundation, popular for creating the Whole Grain Stamp and the Mediterranean Diet Pyramid in 1993 (updated in 2009), made a *"standard shopping check-list"*. If you stick it on the refrigerator, you will be able to check off foods over the week, monitoring when you run out of them or plan meals for the coming days.[42]

Others Mediterranean shopping lists are provided by blog.emeals.com or Dr. Oz's website under Mediterranean Diet Shopping List.[43]

Benefits of the Mediterranean diet

Defining the Mediterranean diet is an important issue. We know there are different ways to define a diet and its pattern. And even when scientists promote similar dietary patterns, some things may vary. For instance we note differences in amounts of foods and nutrients between studies. Therefore it is not wise to investigate the relationship between the Mediterranean diet and health outcomes without a clear definition of the Mediterranean diet.

In fact, we have to admit there are discrepancies between the Mediterranean diet observed and studied today (some important studies are based on a new modified the Mediterranean

---

[42] *Mediterranean diet grocery list*. Oldways Foundation. Retrieved from https://oldwayspt.org/resources/mediterranean-diet-grocery-list
[43] Dr. Oz's Mediterranean Diet Shopping List (2013). Retrieved from https://www.doctoroz.com/article/mediterranean-diet-shopping-list

diet) and the first model based on the Cretan and Southern Italian diets of 1960. Furthermore, in 2018 it may be difficult or expensive in many non-Mediterranean countries to follow the traditional Mediterranean diet. There are also different versions of the Mediterranean diet in Australia and US. What consumers need to know is a universal definition of the Mediterranean diet, calculating an average quantity of foods and nutrients. It makes sense to combine traditional food with some and modern food, when the traditional is not easy to obtain.

It seems useful to identify in a simple way the essential items of a diet.

- Food groups
- Amount of food
- How to cook
- Nutrition

Studies of the different variants of the Mediterranean diet find strong similarities in Food groups (except for the new generation of the Mediterranean diet), and in Nutrition.

There are a few open issues about defining a diet; for instance should a diet be studied on the basis of nutrients rather than of the foods? We know that the public prefers to receive recommendations, which talk about servings of foods rather than about nutrients or grams, but for scientists, there is a distinct advantage to defining the diet by nutrients rather than by foods.

For instance the three famous pyramids tend to show the same general principles, even if some studies vary considerably in

54

the amounts of foods in grams. The variation is less when the nutrient profiles are compared

But there are differences too, in the amount of food per day/week/month for each food group, amounts which can be expressed by

- number of grams for each food groups per day
- number of servings per day/week/month, plus the number of grams of a food group per serving

Another important factor that can generate discrepancies between different diets is how foods are cooked. Boiling and steaming food are the healthiest ways to cook and it is part of the Mediterranean diet. Baking, grilling, roasting, searing, broiling or, of course, frying food are not the healthiest ways.

What role do all these discrepancies have for understanding what works for your brain's health and cognitive functioning? Does the food you are eating preserve your mind or expedite its decline? Scientific studies say that implementing the right food choices is crucial for cognitive health. In fact, despite all difficulties in having equal parameters in the different forms of this diet, scientists were able to identify benefits for the brain's health.

Benefits of the Mediterranean diet

Perlmutter[44] reports that *"in 2007, the journal* Neurology *published a study that looked at more than eight thousand participants who were sixty-five years or older and had totally normal brain functions. The study followed them for up to four years, during which some 280 people developed a form of dementia (most of the 280 were diagnosed with Alzheimer's).*[45] *The researcher aimed to identify patterns in their dietary habits, homing in on their consumption of fish, which contains lots of brain- and heart-healthy omega-3 fats. For people who never consumed fish, the risk of dementia and Alzheimer's disease during the four-year follow-up period was increased by 37 percent. In those individuals who consumed fish on a daily basis, risk for these diseases was reduced by 44 percent. Regular users of butter had no significant change in risk of Alzheimer's, but people, who regularly consumed omega-3-rich oils, such olive, flaxseed, and walnut oil, were 60 percent less likely to develop dementia than those who did not regularly consume such oils. The researchers also found that people who regularly ate omega-6-rich oils – typical in the American diet – but not omega-3-rich oils or fish were twice as likely to develop dementia as people who didn't eat omega-6-rich oils".*

---

[44] Perlmutter D, *Grain brain*, Little, Brown and Company, New York, USA, 2013. P.74

[45] Barberger-Gateau P, Raffaitin C, Letenneur L, Berr C, Tzourio C, Dartigues JF, Alpérovitch A. (2007) Dietary patterns and risk of dementia: the Three-City cohort study. *Neurology.* 13;69(20):1921-30. Retrieved from https://www.ncbi.nlm.nih.gov/pubmed/17998483 DOI:10.1212/01.wnl.0000278116.37320.52

Published studies suggest that greater adherence to the Mediterranean diet is associated with a slower cognitive decline and lower risk of Alzheimer's disease.[46]

According to various epidemiologic studies in the late Nineties, *"dietary fat and energy in old age are high risk factors, while fish and cereals are risk-reduction factors"*[47].

A great number of articles report on the correlation between healthy diets and dementia, but most of them rely on anecdotal evidence and we need researchers to do scientifically controlled experiments. Studies do not prove that the Mediterranean diet prevents brain shrinkage, they show only a proved association.

In fact, scientists of Columbia University (New York) came out with an interesting study.[48] They affirm that eating the Mediterranean diet may affect not only the risk for Alzheimer's disease, (a correlation that has been noted in several earlier studies), but also subsequent disease course.

Although they had already reported that following a Mediterranean style diet was associated with a lower risk of Alzheimer's disease, they never investigated until now whether

[46] Lourida, Ilianna; Soni, Maya; Thompson-Coon, Joanna; Purandare, Nitin; Lang, Iain A.; Ukoumunne, Obioha C.; Llewellyn, David J. (2013) Mediterranean Diet, Cognitive Function, and Dementia: A Systematic Review. *Epidemiology.* Vol. 24 Issue 4 p 479-489 Retrieved from https://journals.lww.com/epidem/Fulltext/2013/07000/Mediterranean_Diet,_Cognitive_Function,_and.1.aspx doi: 10.1097/EDE.0b013e3182944410

[47] Grant WB. (1999). Dietary Links to Alzheimer's Disease: 1999 Update. Journal of Alzheimer's Disease. *Journal of Alzheimer's disease.* 1(4-5):197-201.Retrieved from https://www.ncbi.nlm.nih.gov/pubmed/12214118 PMID: 12214118

[48] Scarmeas N, Luchsinger J A, Mayeux R, and Stern Y. (2007). Mediterranean diet and Alzheimer disease mortality. *Neurology.* 69(11): 1084–1093. Retrieved from https://www.ncbi.nlm.nih.gov/pmc/articles/PMC2673956/ doi: 10.1212/01.wnl.0000277320.50685.7c

this or another diet is associated with the subsequent course and outcome of the disease as compared to the course of the disease in patients following other patterns of diet. Data from this study indicates that a higher adherence to this diet was associated with lower mortality. One of the most exciting findings was that the longer and better Alzheimer's patients follow this diet, the more years they live. In fact, 5 years later only 20% of those with high adherence had died, while the death rate of the intermediate adherence group was double that. In the low adherence diet group, within 5 years, more than half had died, and within 10 years 90% had passed away. And at the end of the study, published for the first time in 2007, the only people still alive were those with a high adherence to the healthiest diet.

Other interesting findings from a study by Harvard University were published in 2012. The relationship between major fat types and cognitive changes were studied in 6,000 healthy, elderly women. The discovery was that a high intake of saturated fats was associated with a poor trajectory of cognition and memory. In fact, women with the highest intake of saturated fats had from 60 to 70% more chance of showing a worsening of brain function. The estimation of cognitive change associated with the consumption of saturated fats was equivalent to about 6 years of aging.[49]

---

[49] Okereke O I, Rosner B A, Kim D H, Kang J H, Cook N R, Manson JA E, Buring J E, Willett W. C, Grodstein F. (2012). Dietary fat types and 4-year cognitive change in community-dwelling older women. Annals of neurology. 72(1): 124–134.   Retrieved   from https://www.ncbi.nlm.nih.gov/pmc/articles/PMC3405188/ doi: 10.1002/ana.23593

According to a randomized trial of the Mediterranean diet pattern for the primary prevention of cardiovascular events,[50] this diet can improve cardiovascular and cognitive health.

A fascinating study[51] compared the incidence of Alzheimer's disease among Nigerian immigrants living in the United States with their relatives who remained in Nigeria. The first one was significantly higher. About this study Perlmutter affirms in his book *"Grain Brain"*[52] that *"all that changed was their environment – specifically their caloric intake. The research clearly focused on the detrimental effects that a higher caloric consumption has on brain health"*. I would consider also the possibility that other neuroprotective lifestyles helped relatives who remained in Nigeria.

In a press statement Yian Gu, one of the authors of another interesting study at Columbia University, affirmed that *"eating at least three to five ounces of fish weekly or eating no more than 3.5 ounces of meat daily may provide considerable protection against loss of brain cells"*. The study[53] was de-

---

[50]Estruch R., Ros E., Salas-Salvadó J., Covas M.-I., Corella D., Arós F., Gómez-Gracia E., Ruiz-Gutiérrez V., Fiol M., Lapetra J., et al. (2013). Primary prevention of cardiovascular disease with a Mediterranean diet. *The New England journal of medicine.* 368(14):1279-90. Retrieved from https://www.ncbi.nlm.nih.gov/pubmed/23432189 doi: 10.1056/NEJMoa1200303

[51] Hendrie HC, Ogunniyi A, Hall KS, Baiyewu O, Unverzagt FW, Gureje O, Gao S, Evans RM, Ogunseyinde AO, Adeyinka AO, Musick B, Hui SL. (2001). Incidence of dementia and Alzheimer disease in 2 Communities: Yoruba residing in Ibadan, Nigeria, and African Americans residing in Indianapolis, Indiana. *JAMA.* 285(6):739-47. Retrieving from https://www.ncbi.nlm.nih.gov/pubmed/11176911

[52] Perlmutter D. (2013). *Grain brain, Little*, Brown and Company, p. 134. New York, USA

[53] Gu Y, Brickman A M, Stern Y, Habeck C G, Razlighi O R, Luchsinger J A, Manly J J, Schupf N, Mayeux R, Scarmeas N. (2015) Mediterranean diet and brain structure in a multiethnic elderly cohort. *Neurology.* 85(20):1744-51. Retrieved from https://www.ncbi.nlm.nih.gov/pubmed/26491085 doi:10.1212/WNL.0000000000002121

signed to *"determine whether higher adherence to a Mediterranean-type diet (MeDi) is related with larger MRI-measured brain volume or cortical thickness"*. The conclusions were that *"among older adults, MeDi adherence was associated with less brain atrophy, with an effect similar to 5 years of aging. Higher fish and lower meat intake might be the 2 key food elements that contribute to the benefits of MeDi on brain structure"*[54].

On the one hand, in recent decades, many trials failed in trying to find an effective pharmacological therapy able to cure Alzheimer's and/or other dementias, on the other hand, in the last years, studies proved how a lifestyle can be effective to prevent or delay symptoms of dementia. And scientific books about them mushroom.

For instance in the book *The End of Alzheimer's*, the author, Dr. Dale E. Bredesen, explains how he can help persons to reverse a cognitive decline, including for those suffering from Alzheimer's. Monitoring *"36 different mechanisms contributing to Alzheimer's disease pathophysiology"*[55] and around 25 lab tests' values makes it possible to understand which of them need to be fixed. In order to do this he "prescribes" a specific diet, and tailored nutritional supplements and drugs. He also suggests daily activities implementing the most important lifestyles healthy for the brain such as regular exercising, sleeping enough and releasing stress.

This book presents a new and interesting paradigm. In fact, after working on the pharmacological approach, scientist proved

---

[54] *Ibid.*
[55] Bredesen D E. (2017). *The End of Alzheimer's,* Avery, Penguin Random House LLC, New York USA.

60

that some non-pharmacological interventions are associated with improved brain functions, some scientists focused their studies on a particular lifestyle to prevent or delay dementia. Later, other scientists started to study the effect of more lifestyles on the brain. Finally, in this book, you can find drugs and healthy lifestyles, in a multi-factor approach because the author recommends concurrently a specific health diet, drugs, nutritional supplements and daily activities associable with lifestyles healthy for the brain.

In July 2017, at the Alzheimer's Association International conference in London, Claire McEvoy, of the University of California, San Francisco's School of Medicine, drawing on the results of four studies, said that the Mediterranean or the similar MIND diet lowered the risk of dementia by a third in those who followed it. These people had better cognitive function and around 30% to 35% lower risk of cognitive impairment during aging. MIND (Mediterranean Intervention for Neurodegenerative Delay) diet was developed by Martha Clare Morris, a Nutritional epidemiologist. Chicago's Rush University Medical Center. MIND diet takes the best brain foods of the Mediterranean diet, including the salt-reducing DASH diet. This is a Mediterranean-DASH Intervention for Neurodegenerative Delay, with DASH standing for Dietary Approaches to Stop Hypertension.

Rudolph Tanzi says, *"Foods that keep blood pressure normal, provide us with antioxidants, and maintain healthy bacteria in our gut, or microbiome, will serve to help keep chronic inflammation in check in the brain and entire body"*.

The neuroscientist Sandrine Thuret[56] said that calorie restriction from 20 to 30% increases neurogenesis, as well intermittent fasting. Some nutrients are efficacious in increasing neurogenesis: flavonoids, contained in dark chocolate or blueberries, or omega-3 fatty acids, present in fatty fish. Conversely a diet rich in high saturated fat has a negative impact on neurogenesis. She also says alcohol decreases neurogenesis, but resveratrol, contained in red wine, promotes survival of new neurons.[57]

Different factors can influence both the onset and the progression of dementia, the dietetic style plays an important role and adherence to the Mediterranean diet has aroused much interest. The intake of large quantities of fruit, vegetables, cereals, nuts and olive oil, and moderate quantities of wine (especially red), fish, white meats and eggs, which characterizes the Mediterranean diet, appears to play a protective role for the brain.

Finally we can list some components of the Mediterranean diet which are particularly healthy:

- Fruits and vegetables: They are rich in antioxidants, protecting the brain from damage caused by oxidative stress, quite common in dementia.
- Dried fruits, in particular nuts and almonds: They are rich in polyunsaturated fatty acids with a protective effect on atherosclerosis.

---

[56] Stangl, D. Thuret, S. (2009). Impact of diet on adult hippocampal neurogenesis. *Genes & nutrition.* 4(4): 271–282.
Retrieved from https://www.ncbi.nlm.nih.gov/pmc/articles/PMC2775886/ doi: 10.1007/s12263-009-0134-5
[57] TED@BCG London. (June 2015). You can grow new brain cells. Here's how. Sandrine Thuret. *TED Institute event in partnership with BCG.* (Video file).
Retrieved from
https://www.ted.com/talks/sandrine_thuret_you_can_grow_new_brain_cells_here_s_how

- Extra-virgin olive oil: It contains many antioxidants, which able to slow the production of toxins in the brain.
- Red wine: Red grape peels are rich in resveratrol, a substance with neuroprotective properties.
- Fish, in particular blue fish: They are rich in omega-3 fatty acids that are among the major components of the cell membrane of the nervous system. Some studies have proposed a reduction of about 60% in the onset of Alzheimer's disease in those who eat a portion of fish at least once a week.[58]

The Mediterranean diet is considered by many scientists as the gold standard in healthy eating. It seems to be effective to prevent many diseases. Scientific studies suggest that the Mediterranean diet increases longevity by lowering cardiovascular disease, inhibiting cancer growth, but also by protecting the body from age-dependent cognitive decline. It helps to get and stay at your ideal weight, control your blood sugar, and improve your bone and brain health.

High consumption of dietary fiber, low glycemic index and glycemic load, anti-inflammatory effects, and antioxidant compounds may act together to produce these favorable effects on health status.[59]

---

[58] Fondazione Dieta Mediterranea. *La dieta mediterranea contro la demenza e il morbo di Alzheimer.* Retrieved from https://www.fondazionedietamediterranea.it/ricerca-2/gli-effetti-benefici-della-dieta/la-dieta-mediterranea-contro-la-demenza-e-il-morbo-di-alzheimer/

[59]Farooqui T, Farooqui A A. (2017) *Role of the Mediterranean Diet in the Brain and Neurodegenerative Diseases*, Academic Press, San Diego, California, USA.

Scientific evidence also links the Mediterranean diet to stronger bones, a healthier heart and longer life, along with a reduced risk for diabetes and high blood pressure.

IV

APPENDIX

An Italian Case Study

How can we measure the impact of educating persons about their own health on lifestyles?

How long should a person follow a new lifestyle before it can be considered a new, acquired lifestyle?

From 2005 to 2007, in Italy, as executive at Regional Agency for Healthcare Puglia, I personally ran a program about healthy lifestyles. We identified some experts in the field to provide to General Practitioners (GPs, same as Family doctors) with the last scientific evidence about healthy lifestyles. Other experts taught to GPs how to educate patients about health lifestyles in 10 minutes in their own ambulatory patients who got into it.

The GPs would start the meeting with a 10-questions questionnaire which aimed at assessing their lifestyle: physical activity or diet. Later, during this same meeting, using a communication protocol, the GPs were instructed to teach patients, in 10 minutes, why it makes sense to change their lifestyle and how to go about it. The 10 minutes were a true educational

65

talk. They would follow up with their patients during a timeframe of from three months.

The most important issue for me was to measure education's effectiveness on lifestyles. The Italian Continuing Medical Education (CME)[60] Program neither required nor provided a way to measure its efficacy. On the contrary my approach could show how the program achieved its goals. In the program, therefore, I wanted to convert the National Educational Goals into educational impact indicators or educational effectiveness. In this way I gave to the program an objective measurement system, an indicators' set.

My methodological intuition was as trivial as it was pioneering. Trivial as to intuition, pioneering as to implementation. At that time everyone was talking about quality in CME Program (and today they are still talking), but no one had or has ever really implemented a system to demonstrate, with the use of data, the effectiveness of CME for people's health. This step, elementary but essential, was perhaps decisive in the recognition by the Italian CME Program's Committee[61] of the nature and the title of a trial.

Maybe this approach was the key to obtaining the highest number of credits-hours up to that time ever had in an Italian CME Program: 2.5 credits per hour, 40 credits for 16 hours. In 2005, credits' national average was 0.7 per hour, in a range between 0.5-1.25.

---

[60] *Educazione continua in medicina (ECM)* is the Italian national program of Continuing Medical Education. Started in 2002, it is mandatory for all health professionals with the aim of keeping up-to-date and competent.
[61] This committee organizes and controls all the activities

The GPs were not required to educate a minimum number of persons to get CME credits. For this reason, the data could be considered true and reliable; they were not molded by the opportunity of getting many CME credits. The only reason for attending this program would be to know more about healthy lifestyles from a group of experts or to test a new educational method.

The program was planned in this sequence.

- GPs attended an 8-hours' class.
- GPs had 60 days to meet patients on the job, in their clinic, where they performed the "health education's communicative protocol".
- GPs attended a 4-hours meeting to discuss how effective was that protocol (assessment of educational impact).
- GPs had 90 days to follow up in their clinic with the patients previously educated. This was needed to verify possible changes in lifestyles. The assessment of educational impact was performed on the job.
- GPs attended a 4-hour meeting to discuss how patients complied with healthy lifestyles and how the program was effective to change lifestyles.

It was essential to my understanding of lifestyle change to have an objective measurement. This is the list of questions about health. The list was suggested from dr. Ettore Samele, nutritional biologist. For every "yes", the persons achieve the score at the side.

Lifestyle Questionnaire

Answer the questions and add the points
assigned to each question

1.	Do you check your weight at least once a month?	5
2.	Do you consume at least 5 portions of vegetables and/or fruits each day?	10
3.	Do you drink at least 1 liter and a half of water a day?	5
4.	Do you drink no more than 2-3 glasses of wine a day? (2 for females and 3 for males)	5
5.	Do you use only extra virgin olive oil as a condiment (cooked-raw)?	10
6.	Do you consume more fish than meat during the week?	7
7.	Do you read nutrition labels?	5
8.	Do you have breakfast daily?	10
9.	Did you reduce consumption of salt added during the meals?	7
10.	Do you walk at least an hour a day?	7
11.	Do you have at least three meals a day?	5

For this questionnaire, the highest score achievable was 79.

- A score between 60 and 79, excellent quality in lifestyle
- A score between 40 and 59, adequate quality in lifestyle
- A score between 0 and 39, poor quality in lifestyle

The educational goals of this program matched with the following two goals from among those listed by Italian CME Program's Committee:

- Health education (for people)
- Improvement of healthy lifestyles

I found these two following indicators as the most important for the community:

- the number of citizens, who received 10 minutes' education from GPs about health lifestyle (physical activity or diet) .
- the number of citizens, who improved their healthy lifestyle after 10 minutes' education.

I started to work on this program in 2005, ending it in 2007. Eleven out of 12 involved PHCs (Public Healthcare Companies) of the region of Puglia participated.

The final data represented for me the most rewarding result.

Number of districts in the 11 involved PHCs	45
Number of GPs in the 11 PHCs	3,122
Number of GPs signed up for this program	1,770
Number of GPs signed up for this program, who then attended all educational sessions	1,358
Percentage of GPs signed up for this program compared to total number of GPs in the 11 PHCs	56.9%
Percentage of GPs who attended all educational sessions compared to total number of GPs in the 11 PHCs	44.4%
Percentage of GPs who attended all educational sessions compared to all GPs signed for the program	78%
Number of times the course was offered	50
Number of patients seen by GPs enrolled in the program	41,848
Number of patients who received 10 minutes' education from GPs about healthy lifestyle (physical activity or diet)	**24,371**
Number of patients seen by GPs in the program who already complied with correct physical activity or a healthy diet	5,318
Number of follow up with patients who received education from GPs.	**21,713**
Number of patients who received education about physical activity or diet and improved their lifestyle, based on following check.	**14,378**
Percentage of patients who improved their lifestyle among those followed up by GPs	**66.2%**

70

BIBLIOGRAPHY

Alterra, A. (2007) *The Caregiver A life with Alzheimer's*. Ithaca, NYS, USA: Cornell University Press.

Ertel, A.K. Glymour, M.M. Berkman L.F. (2007). Effects of Social Integration on Preserving Memory Function in a Nationally Representative US Elderly Population American. *Journal of Public Health*. vol. 98, pp. 1215-1220

Balducci C., Melchiorre M.G., Quattrini S., Lamura G., (2008). Prendersi cura di un familiare affetto da demenza: evidenze da uno studio cross-sectional sul carico sostenuto e sul benessere psicologico del caregiver. *Quaderni europei sul nuovo welfare*. Quaderno n. 10/2008.

Beach, S.R. Schulz, R. Yee, J.L. Jackson S. (2000) Negative and positive health effects of caring for a disabled spouse: Longitudinal findings from the Caregiver Health Effects Study. *Psychology and aging*. 15(2): 259-71. Retrieved from https://www.ncbi.nlm.nih.gov/pubmed/10879581

Bredesen, D. (2017). *The end of Alzheimer's*. New York, USA: Penguin Random House LLC.

Chopra, D., Tanzi, R. (2018). *The Healing self*. New York, USA: Harmony books.

Christakis, N.A. Allison, P.D. (2006). Mortality after the hospitalization of a spouse. *The New England journal of medi-*

cine. 354 (7) 719-30. Retrieved from https://www.ncbi.nlm.nih.gov/pubmed/16481639

Colombari, C.M. (2009). *Ho sognato uno spazio morbido*. Torino, Italy: Antigone edizioni.

Manuale per prendersi cura del malato di Alzheimer. (3rd edit.) (2006). Commissione Europea Alzheimer's Europe. Milano, Italy.

Rice, R. (2000). *Manual of Home Health Nursing Procedures*. St. Louis, Missouri, USA: Mosby.

Coon D.W., Gallagher-Thompson D., Thompson L.W., (2003). *Innovative Interventions to Reduce Caregiver Distress: a Clinical Guide*. New York, NY, USA: Springer Publishing Company, Inc.

Farran, C.J. Staffileno, B.A. Gilley, D.W. McCann J.J. Yan Li, Castro, C.M., King A.C. (2008). A Lifestyle Physical Activity Intervention for Caregivers of Persons With Alzheimer's Disease, *American Journal of Alzheimer's Disease and Other Dementias*, 23(2): 132, 142, College of Nursing, Chicago.

Fletcher K., Dementia, in Capezuti E., Zwicker D., Mezey M., Fulmer T. (2008). Evidence- based geriatric nursing protocols for best practice. (3rd ed.) pp. 83-109. New York (NY) USA: Springer Publishing Company.

Farooqui, T., Farooqui A. A. (2017). *Role of the Mediterranean Diet in the Brain and Neurodegenerative Diseases*. California, USA: Academic Press, San Diego.

73

Gallagher-Thompson D., Thompson L.W., (2008). *Treating Late Life Depression: A Cognitive- Behavioral Therapy Approach, Therapist Guide*. New York, USA: Oxford University Press.

Gardini, N. (2007). *Lo sconosciuto*. Milano, Italy: Alpha Test.

Given, B. Given, C.W. Stommel, M. et al. (1994) Predictors of use of secondary careers used by the elderly following hospital discharge. *Journal of Aging and Health*. 6(3): 353-76. Retrieved from http://journals.sagepub.com/doi/abs/10.1177/089826439400600305

Given, C.W. Stommel, M. Given, B. Osuch, J. Kurtz, M.E. Kurtz, J.C. (1993) The influence of the cancer patient's symptoms, functional states on patient's depression and family caregiver's reaction and depression. *Health psychology: official journal of the Division of Health Psychology, American Psychological Association*. 12(4): 277-85. Retrieved from https://www.ncbi.nlm.nih.gov/pubmed/8404801

Green, L.W., Ottoson, J.M. (1999). *Community and Population Health*. Boston, (MA), USA: WCB McGraw Hill.

Grutzner, H. (2001). Alzheimer's, A Caregiver's Guide and Sourcebook. NY, USA: Wiley.
Jelloun, T.B. (2007). *Mia madre, la mia bambina*. Torino, Italy: Einaudi.

Kurtz, M.E. Given, B. Kurtz, J.C. Given, C.W. (1994). The interaction of age, symptoms, and survival status on physical and mental health of patients with cancer and their families. *Cancer.* 74 (7 Suppl.): 2071-8. Retrieved from https://www.ncbi.nlm.nih.gov/pubmed/8087774

Laidlaw, K. Thompson, L.W. Gallagher Thompson, D. Dick-Siskin L. (2003). *Cognitive Behavior Therapy With Older People.* Hoboken, NJ, USA: John Wiley & Sons Ltd.

Leahy W., Fuzy, J. Grafe, J. (2004). *Providing Home Care.* Albuquerque, NM, USA: Hartman Publishing, Inc.

Lee P.R., Estes C.L. Rodriguez, F. M (2003). *The Nation's Health.* Sudbury, MA, USA: Jones and Bartlett Pub.

Levkoff, S.E. Chen H., Fisher J. McIntyre J. (2006). *Evidence Based Behavioral Health Practices for Older Adults.* New York, NY, USA: Springer Publishing Company.

Lichtenberg P.A., Murman D.L., Mellow A.M. (2003). Handbook of Dementia. Hoboken, NJ, US: John Wiley & Sons Inc.

Mace, N.L. Rabins, P. (2001). *The 36 Hour Day.* New York USA: Warner Books.

McCurry, S.M. (2006). *When a Family Member Has Dementia: Steps to Becoming a Resilient Caregiver.* Westport, CT, USA: Praeger Publisher.

Morone, J.A. Litman, T.J. Robins, L.S. (2008). *Health Politics and Policy.* Clifton Park, New York, USA: Delmar Publishers.

75

Murphy, J. Carrol, A. (2003). *Nursing Homes and Alternatives: What New York Families Need to Know.* New York, USA: FRIA.

Naylor, M.D. (2002). Transitional care of older adults. *Annual review of nursing research.* 20:127-47. Retrieved from https://www.ncbi.nlm.nih.gov/pubmed/12092508

Noto, V. (2003). *Il Manuale di ausili e cure del paziente geriatrico a domicilio.* Torino, Italy: UTET.

Perlmutter, D. (2013). *Grain brain.* New York, USA: Little, Brown and Company.

Gainotti, G. Provinciali, L, Scarpino, O. Trabucchi, M. *Malattia di Alzheimer: manuale per gli operatori.* Milano, Italy: F.Angeli.

Reinhard, S.C. Given, B. Petlick, H.N. Bemis, A. (2008). Chapter 14. Supporting Family Caregivers in Providing Care. *Patient Safety and Quality: An evidence- Based Handbook for Nurses.* Hughes RG, editor. Rockville (MD): Agency for Healthcare Research and Quality (USA).

Rice, R. (2000). *Manual of Home Health Nursing Procedures.* St. Louis, Missouri, USA: Mosby.

Ritchie, K. Touchon, J. Ledèsert, B. (1998). Mixed cognitive and affective disorders in elderly: A longitudinal study of related disability. *Archives of gerontology and geriatrics.* Vol. 26, suppl. 1, 443-450. Retrieved from https://www.sciencedirect.com/science/article/pii/S016749439 880065

Robinson, J. Curry, L. Gruman, C. Porter, M. Henderson, C. Pillemer, K. Partners in care giving in a special care environment: Cooperative communication between staff and families in dementia units. *The Gerontologist*. Vol. 47, n. 4 pp. 504-515. Retrieved from https://www.ncbi.nlm.nih.gov/pubmed/17766671

Sacks, O. (1998). *The Man Who Mistook His Wife For a Hat*. New York, USA: Touchstone.

Salza, C. (2007). *Arteterapia e Alzheimer*. Como, Italy: Nodo Libri.

Schulz, R. Beach S.R. (1999). *Caregiving as a risk factor for mortality: The caregiver health effects study. JAMA.* 282(23): 2215-9. Retrieved from https://www.ncbi.nlm.nih.gov/pubmed/10605972

Schulz, R. Beach, S.R. Lind, B. et al. (2001). Involvement in caregiving and adjustment to death of a spouse: Findings from the Caregiver Health Effects Study. *JAMA.* 285(24):3123-9. Retrieved from https://www.ncbi.nlm.nih.gov/pubmed/11427141

Shenk, D. (2003). *The Forgetting Alzheimer's: Portrait of an Epidemic*. New York, USA: Anchor Book.

Tsai, S. Arnold R.M. (2007). Prognostication in Dementia #150. *Journal of Palliative Medicine.* Vol. 10, No.3. Retrieved from https://doi.org/10.1089/jpm.2007.9949

Sörensen, S. Pinquart, M. Duberstein, P. (2002). How Effective Are Interventions With Caregivers? An Updated Meta-Analysis. *The Gerontologist.* 42(3):356-372. Retrieved from https://www.ncbi.nlm.nih.gov/pubmed/12040138 PMID: 12040138

Sorocco, H.K. Lauderdale, S. (2011). *Handbook of Behavioral and Cognitive Therapies with Older Adults.* New York, (NY) USA: Springer.

Spreen, O. Strauss E. (1998). *A Compendium of Neuro Psychological Tests: Administration, norms and commentary.* New York, (NY) USA: Oxford University Press.

Strauss, C. J. (2002). *Talking to Alzheimer's.* Chicago, (IL) USA: New Hambirger Publications.

Sultz, H. Young K.M. (1997). *Health Care USA - Understanding Its Organization and Delivery.* Frederick, MD, USA: Aspen Publishers Inc.

The Alzheimer's activities guide. (2005). NY, NY, USA: Forest Laboratories.

Tideiksar, R. (2002). *Falls in older people: prevention and management.* Baltimore, MD, USA: Health Professions Press.

Vigorelli, P. (2008). *Alzheimer's senza paura*. Milano, Italy: Rizzoli.

Warner M.L., (2005). *In search of the Alzheimer's Wanderer: A workbook to protect your loved one*. Ashland, OH, USA: Purdue University Press.

Yeo, G. Gallagher-Thompson D. (1996). Ethnicity and the Dementias, USA: Routledge/Taylor & Francis Group. New York, NY, US.